SOCIAL JUSTICE, EQUALITY AND EMPOWERMENT

AF848794

URBAN SLUMS AND THE SOCIAL PRODUCTION OF INFANT MORTALITY RATES IN THE LESS DEVELOPED COUNTRIES: A MACRO-COMPARATIVE, QUANTITATIVE ANALYSIS

SOCIAL JUSTICE, EQUALITY AND EMPOWERMENT

Additional books in this series can be found on Nova's website under the Series tab.

Additional E-books in this series can be found on Nova's website under the E-book tab.

SOCIAL JUSTICE, EQUALITY AND EMPOWERMENT

URBAN SLUMS AND THE SOCIAL PRODUCTION OF INFANT MORTALITY RATES IN THE LESS DEVELOPED COUNTRIES: A MACRO-COMPARATIVE, QUANTITATIVE ANALYSIS

JAMES RICE

NOVINKA

Nova Science Publishers, Inc.
New York

For permission to use material from this book please contact us:
Telephone 631-231-7269; Fax 631-231-8175
Web Site: http://www.novapublishers.com

Additional color graphics may be available in the e-book version of this book.

LIBRARY OF CONGRESS CATALOGING-IN-PUBLICATION DATA

Rice, James.
Urban slums and the social production of infant mortality rates in the less developed countries : a macro-comparative, quantitative analysis / James Rice.
p. cm.
Includes index.
ISBN 978-1-61761-314-2 (softcover)
1. Infants--Mortality--Developing countries. 2. Slums--Developing countries. 3. Cities and towns--Developing countries. I. Title.
HB1323.I42D448 2010
305.23209172'4--dc22

2010031455

Published by Nova Science Publishers, Inc. † New York

CONTENTS

PREFACE

We utilize first-difference panel regression analysis to assess the direct effect of urban slum prevalence or the proportion of the total population living in urban slum conditions on national level measures of infant mortality rates over the period 1990 to 2005. Utilizing data on 81 less developed countries, the results illustrate increasing urban slum prevalence over the period is a robust predictor of increasing infant mortality rates. This effect obtains net the statistically significant influence of gross domestic product per capita, fertility rate, and female secondary school enrollment. The results confirm urban slum prevalence growth is an important contextual dynamic whereby the social production of infant mortality is enacted in the less developed countries. This is congruent with the meta-theoretical assumption derived from social epidemiology suggesting the built environment has a recognizable influence on social processes; and it highlights, moreover, the importance of focusing upon the contradictions of urban social organization in order to more fully conceptualize the social determinants of health and illness in the less developed countries.

Chapter 1

INTRODUCTION

Slums have long been a dimension of the urban landscape and the basic features of slum life have changed little over time; what has changed in recent decades is the increasing depth and magnitude of urban slum conditions in the less developed countries (United Nations Population Fund [UNFPA] 2007). The "concentrated disadvantage" (Vlahov et al. 2007: i16) characteristic of many urban slums, moreover, constitutes an increasingly prominent structural characteristic shaping population-level patterns of health and illness.

Worldwide the aggregate urban slum population grew 39 percent over the period 1990-2005 (United Nations Human Settlements Programme [UN-HABITAT] 2008). Currently the one billion individuals living in urban slum conditions comprise roughly one-third of the world's total urban population, 43 percent of the urban population in the developing countries, and 78 percent of the urban population in the poorest, least developed countries (UN-HABITAT 2003a, 2006). Recent projections suggest the overall urban slum population worldwide is projected to increase steadily in the coming decades by an estimated 27 million new slum residents annually from 2000-2020 (UN-HABITAT 2003a).

The remarkable growth of urban slums in recent decades is a reflection of the increasing urbanization of poverty; such reorganization gives form to evolving "risk spaces" (Fitzpatrick and LaGory 2000: 12) or areas in which a sub-population is disproportionately subject to a myriad of hazards relative to other segments of society. In stark contrast to the generally beneficial health consequences of urban social organization, urban slum conditions are increasingly characterized by an observable "urban penalty." Indeed, urban slum areas often exhibit poorer health outcomes, lower life expectancy rates, lower levels of education, and diminished economic opportunities relative to non-slum urban populations (UN-HABITAT 2006). The assertion that urban children are healthier than children in rural areas is increasingly in doubt, moreover, given the deteriorating living conditions of many urban settlements (Bartlett 2003). Child malnutrition within urban slums is often comparable to that observed in rural areas and the incidence of waterborne diseases and respiratory illnesses is generally higher (UN-HABITAT 2006).

Within the social science research literature the empirical examination of the socio-spatial health disparities characteristic of an urban penalty is predominantly focused on variation in health outcomes across slum and non-slum areas of a particular city under examination. The present study approaches the empirical evaluation of the urban penalty from a different unit of analysis. We develop and test the proposition that urban slum prevalence or proportion of the total population living in urban slum conditions has a recognizable effect measured at the national level.

Drawing from social epidemiology as an overarching meta-theoretical framework, we argue the magnitude and depth of urban slum conditions in the LDCs is now so pronounced as to constitute a key structural characteristic shaping inequalities in health and illness viewed from a macro-comparative, cross-national scale. The built urban environment is not simply a reflection of or container for social organizational patterns but a key dimension shaping variant risk spaces and the social production of morbidity and mortality--particularly as it concerns the well-being of the most vulnerable members of a population. Infant mortality rates in the developing countries, in turn, are not simply the consequence of individual-level risk factors, as suggested by the dominant biomedical model, but also socially produced within the contextual, substandard living conditions characteristic of urban slums.

First-difference panel regression utilizing ordinary least squares (OLS) estimation is employed to assess the degree to which urban slum prevalence growth over the period 1990 to 2005 is a statistically significant predictor of increasing infant mortality rates over the period. We also engage in cross-sectional OLS regression as a sensitivity check to further evaluate the impact of urban slum prevalence on infant mortality rates employing an alternative control variable not available in the panel analysis due to data availability restrictions.

The growth of urban slums, of note, is a trend that has gone largely unnoticed by social scientists employing a quantitative, macro-comparative research approach examining health disparities in the LDCs;[1] this is problematic as managing urban growth in a manner that broadly capitalizes on the advantages of urbanization, while minimizing the liabilities, is an increasingly important development objective (Cohen 2006). Attainment of the Millennium Development Goals (MDGs), benchmarks established by the United Nations member states in 2000, is predicated in part upon improving the living conditions of urban slum residents in the developing countries. As Moreno and Warah (2006) note, they are the second largest target group, after rural populations, in need of development aid; working to improve the living conditions of urban slum residents, in turn, will significantly enhance progress towards meeting a majority of the MDGs (Moreno and Warah 2006). This fact is recognized in particular in MDG 7, Target 11, which endeavors: "By 2020, to have achieved a significant improvement in the lives of at least 100 million slum-dwellers." This is a notable goal, but if current trends continue there will be over 500 million additional urban slum residents worldwide in 2020 than when the MDGs were originally established in 2000.[2]

---

[1] Reliable comparative data on urban slum conditions in the LDCs only became available with the publication of a series of UN-HABITAT reports in 2003 (UN-HABITAT 2003a, 2003b) and updated periodically in subsequent years. This data collection effort is in response to the creation of the United Nations Millennium Development Goals (MDGs).

[2] This estimate is based on current annual urban slum growth worldwide extrapolated to 2020. For current estimates of annual urban slum growth see UN-HABITAT (2003a).

Chapter 2

URBAN SLUMS IN THE LESS DEVELOPED COUNTRIES

A slum constitutes, in general terms, a densely populated area exhibiting substandard housing and standard of living (UN-HABITAT 2003b). In concrete terms, Table 1 outlines the criteria established by UN-HABITAT to delineate slum versus non-slum urban populations. The definition focuses on the physical and legal dimensions of urban residence as designation is based on the absence of one or more of the following: improved water supply, improved sanitation, sufficient living area, durability of construction, and security of tenure. [1]

The degree of deprivation is predicated on how many of the criteria highlighted in Table 1 are absent. Lack of access to improved water and sanitation are the most common indicators of urban slum residence in the developing countries (UN-HABITAT 2003a). Lack of durability of construction and overcrowding are the next most common indicators. Approximately one-fifth of slums worldwide are extremely deprived as indicated by the absence of three or more of the established standards (UN-HABITAT 2007a).

---

[1] Security of tenure is recognized as a dimension of slum residence but does not currently constitute an aspect of urban slum measurement at the cross-national level due to insufficient data (see UN-HABITAT 2003a: 50-51).

Table 1. Criteria for delineating slum and non-slum urban households

An urban household is defined as a slum dwelling if it lacks one or more of the following:
1. *Access to an Improved Water Supply*--that provides a sufficient quantity of water for family use (at least 20 liters/person/day), at an affordable price (less than 10% of total household income), without requiring extreme effort to obtain (less than one hour a day for the minimum sufficient quantity). In addition, an improved water supply consists of the following delivery systems: • Piped connection to house or plot • Public stand pipe serving no more than 5 households • Bore hole • Protected dug well • Protected spring • Rain water collection
2. *Access to Improved Sanitation*--consisting of a private or public toilet shared between a reasonable numbers of people. Improved sanitation consists of the following services: • Direct connection to public sewer • Direct connection to a septic tank • Pour flush latrine • Ventilated pit latrine
3. *Sufficient Living Area.* Overcrowding is defined as 3 or more people per habitable room (minimum of four square meters of space).
4. *Durability of Construction.* A dwelling is defined as durable if it is built in a non-hazardous location and exhibits structural qualities adequate to protect its inhabitants from the extremes of climatic conditions, including rain, heat, cold, and humidity. A non-hazardous location is defined as: • The dwelling is not located on or near toxic waste • The dwelling is not located in a flood plain • The dwelling is not located on a steep slope • The dwelling is not located in a dangerous right of way (rail, highway, airport, power lines) Assessment of structural quality is shaped by prevailing local conditions and therefore exhibits considerable variability in definition. An earthen floor, for example, may be defined as durable in some countries but un-durable in other countries relative to broader prevailing living conditions. An underlying criterion, in turn, for assessing durability of construction is the degree to which a dwelling exhibits a permanency of structure in terms of the walls, roof, and floor in manner that protects it inhabitants from the weather without need for major repair.
5. *Security of Tenure*--residents have protection against arbitrary and/or unlawful eviction.

Table adapted from UN-HABITAT (2003a, 2003b).

The designation "improved" refers to water and sanitation provisioning that meet one of several criteria. The standards measure both quantity and source protection of drinking water and the degree to which sanitation facilities reduce the chances of individuals coming into contact with human excreta and thereby a common pathway of disease transmission. Durability of construction refers to the materials utilized and the location in which the household is situated relative to common hazards found in the urban biophysical and built environment. Deficient housing complicates water, sanitation, and food preparation and storage needs (Brown 2003). Further, urban slum residents often occupy the most marginalized and least economically productive land and therefore live coincident to a number of geologic and industrial hazards thereby increasing exposure to floods, landslides, and pollution (Davis 2006; Satterthwaite 1993).

Sufficient living area is of concern as overcrowding makes adequate hygienic practices to maintain health increasingly problematic. Overcrowding makes urban residents vulnerable to a litany of communicable diseases that include tuberculosis, acute respiratory infections, and meningitis (Sclar et al. 2005). The higher prevalence of malnutrition within urban slums, moreover, facilitates the transmission of illness due to lowered immunity among slum populations (Sclar et al. 2005).

Security of tenure refers to the degree to which residents are protected against arbitrary and/or unlawful eviction (UN-HABITAT 2003b). Many slum households do not hold formal legal title to the land upon which they reside or legally enforceable agreements constituting proof of tenure arrangements (UN-HABITAT 2003a, 2003b). Frequently slums consist of illegally or informally occupied areas of land (Bolay 2006; Davis 2006; UN-HABITAT 2003a, 2003b). Many are characterized by an uncertain and precarious existence as eviction is an ever-present threat and there exist, in turn, substantial disincentives to individual and community investment in upgrading living conditions (Bolay 2006).

Chapter 3

THE BUILT URBAN ENVIRONMENT AND THE SOCIAL PRODUCTION OF INFANT MORTALITY

Social epidemiology is a specialized branch of epidemiology focusing on the social-organizational production of disproportionate illness among disadvantaged segments of a population (Berkman and Kawachi 2000; Cwikel 2006; Krieger 2001a, 2001b; Link and Phelan 1996; Oakes and Kaufman 2006).[1] Social epidemiology frequently adopts an individual-level unit of analysis but is increasingly embracing a population-level perspective (Macintyre and Ellaway 2000); this entails an effort to examine the socio-organizational patterns and large-scale structural arrangements that influence the health outcomes of a defined population. In turn, this often necessitates the consideration of poverty, discrimination, and various forms of inequality within society as factors impacting differential morbidity and mortality rates (Krieger 1999; Link and Phelan 1996; Turshen 1977).

The recognition that social factors shape health and illness has a long history (Cassel 1964; Engels 1968 [1845]; Yankauer 1950) and yet social epidemiology is a relatively new and often contested branch of epidemiology as it challenges the overly narrow and "desocialized" biomedical model focusing upon individual-level biological and behavioral risk factors

---

[1] Medical sociology and social epidemiology both include a focus on the social determinants of variant patterns of health and illness and both borrow from and inform the other. We use the term "social epidemiology" in a broad, general sense which also recognizes the insights and contributions of medical sociologists.

(Berkman and Kawachi 2000; Farmer 1999; Farmer et al. 2006; Krieger 2000). The biomedical model investigates why a particular individual is sick whereas social epidemiology involves inquiry into the societal dynamics shaping *susceptibility to* rather than the biomedical *mechanisms of* disease causation (Krieger 2001a, 2001b).

The objective of social epidemiology is to document the manner in which "societies shape patterns of disease" (Link and Phelan 1996: 471; Waitzkin 1981). Such insights are more provocatively conceptualized as "structural violence" (Farmer 1999, 2004, Farmer et al. 2006; Galtung 1969, 1990). Recognizing that overt and episodic violence is but one aspect of the injury suffered by the poor and marginalized, structural violence refers to the inequitable social structural and institutional patterns that predominantly disadvantage particular groups in society. Galtung (1969) argues embedded, systematic patterns that inhibit the fulfillment of basic needs of some members of society are less easily recognizable than direct violence and yet are more stable and durable; Farmer (1999, 2004) further notes that structural violence is expressed as individual level pathology and population level disparities in morbidity and mortality. Arguably, structural violence underlies the remarkable expansion of urban slums in the developing countries in recent decades and the inadequate built urban environment is increasingly the site of the social production of disparities in health and illness in the developing countries.

The Influence of the Built Urban Environment on Infant Mortality Rates

The built environment consists of the "tangible settings which people create for repeated use" (Dunlap, Michelson, and Stalker 2001: 1) and "that part of the environment constructed by human intention and effort" (Kilmartin 2001: 167). The inadequate built urban environment arguably has a direct, though not deterministic, influence on health disparities that is not synonymous with or reducible to invocations of "urbanization" or "poverty." It is an expression of prevailing social and economic organization and, in turn, the social production of uneven health and illness. Socio-economic processes contribute to the formation of urban slum conditions but it is the dilapidated, semi-permanent built urban environment in which inequities in health and illness are increasingly enacted. This proposition, in turn, rests upon the meta-theoretical assumption that the built and biophysical environment has cognitive, behavioral, and physiological impacts discernable at the individual and population level (Dunlap and Catton 1979).

Poverty, overcrowding, malnutrition, insufficient garbage disposal, lack of adequate water drainage, and unsafe drinking water and sanitation coalesce around the social organization of marginalized populations in urban slums. The inadequate built urban environment within many developing countries, therefore, constitutes a key barrier to progressive social wellbeing and even a catalyst of retrogression; this may be particularly the case for children (Bartlett 2003; Satterthwaite 1993). The five illnesses at the root of a majority of child deaths in the developing countries include pneumonia, diarrhea, malaria, measles, and HIV/AIDS (UN-HABITAT 2007b). Each is prevalent in many urban slums due to substandard living conditions and overcrowding (UN-HABITAT 2007b). Inadequate access to clean water and sanitation, in particular, are a direct cause of a substantial proportion of deaths of infants annually (UNDP 2006). Poor water quality and quantity and inadequate sanitation are linked to a number of waterborne and water-washed diseases (UNDP 2006).

Greater morbidity and mortality among urban slum infants is not simply the consequence of household level deficiencies but also includes health issues arising within the context of the broader slum settlement (Agarwal and Taneja 2005; Awasthi and Agarwal 2003; Bartlett 2003). Inadequate water drainage and waste removal often creates areas of contamination extending throughout the surrounding community (Bartlett 2003); many slums lack safe places for children to play outdoors (Bartlett 2003; Satterthwaite 1993), and there is litany of indoor and outdoor chemical pollutants frequently encountered in low-income urban areas that compromise the health of children (Satterthwaite 1993). Although they often border and even roughly encircle urban areas, moreover, in general slums are socially, politically, and economically isolated from the broader urban setting and their residents lack access to many formal institutions in society (UN-HABITAT 2003b). There are frequently considerable barriers to accessing quality health care and emergency services for slum residents (Sclar et al. 2005).

Micro and meso-level medical science research indeed illustrates that infants residing in urban slums are subject to a litany of diseases. Neonatal mortality, or death within the first 28 days, is commonplace in many urban slums and is generally preceded by sepsis, perinatal asphyxia, and prematurity (Fernandez, Mondkar, and Mathai 2003; Vaid et al. 2007). Beyond the neonatal period infants residing in urban slums frequently die of diarrheal disease and respiratory infections (Vaid et al. 2007); high rates of diarrheal disease, in particular, is a stark reflection of the lack of clean drinking water and adequate sanitation facilities (Fotso et al. 2007; Vaid et al. 2007).

Home births and births not accompanied by a trained medical professional are also commonplace in many urban slums (Fernandez et al. 2003; Gulati and Jaswal 1998; Hoque and Selwyn 1996; Rahi et al. 2006); this contributes to late recognition of neonatal illness, inadequate antenatal care, and delays in seeking appropriate medical services (Fernandez et al. 2003). Further, many slum children are malnourished, increasing their susceptibility to illness (Bartlett 2003; Ghosh and Shah 2004; Wagstaff et al. 2004). Research illustrates children living in urban slums in India, for example, are more malnourished than non-slum urban and even rural children (Ghosh and Shah 2004). Malnourishment among mothers, in addition, contributes to low-birth weight neonates and, therefore, a key risk factor for increased infant death (Fernandez et al. 2003).

Despite the established medical science literature substantiating the risks to infant health of urban slum living conditions, the macro-comparative research approach has yet to empirically focus on the inadequate built urban environment and infant mortality rates in the developing countries. We argue this is potentially problematic as conceptualizing the influence of urban slum conditions on infant mortality rates can contribute to the identification of the upstream, population-level challenges to public health improvement in the developing countries. As McKinlay (1981) notes, a majority of resources and attention devoted to public health concerns are applied downstream or in reference to problem-solving interventions designed to address various, and shifting, issues. Often the real and more enduring problems, however, exist upstream in terms of access to and adequacy of health care provisioning and the social and environmental context in which different segments of a population reside, thus shaping differential exposure to risk (McKinlay 1981). Arguably health and illness is shaped, in part, through the suitability of the built urban environment--a dynamic not reducible to individual-level biological and behavioral risk factors nor adequately addressed through downstream medical interventions alone.

Chapter 4

METHODOLOGY

We utilize first-difference panel regression with OLS estimation to analyze the effect of the change in urban slum prevalence on change in infant mortality rates over the period 1990-2005 among LDCs with available data. We also include additional predictor variables illustrated to have a strong, robust effect on infant mortality rates as identified through previous macro-comparative research. Given that data is unavailable for a key control variable, we also engage in cross-sectional OLS regression as a sensitivity check to further evaluate the statistical significance and stability of urban slum prevalence on infant mortality rates in 2007.

Examination of the period 1990-2005 is predicated upon the longest span of time for which comparable data on the dependent variable is currently available. We define LDCs as consisting of non-high income countries as designated by the World Bank for 1990 (World Bank 2006). The countries included in the regression analyses are listed in Table 1A in the Appendix. To maximize available data we use listwise deletion and allow the number of countries to vary between regression models. We incorporate into the analysis countries that possess a minimum population of one million to avoid anomalies related to low population countries. Based on data availability, the tested models range from 81-78 countries. Of note, urban slum prevalence data for eastern European countries is unavailable for 1990 and therefore the analysis presented does not include any developing countries from this region.

In a first difference model change in the dependent variable over time is regressed on change in the independent variables over the same time period (Babones 2009; Finkel 1995; Firebaugh and Beck 1994; Jackman 1980; Liker, Augustyniak, and Duncan 1985). This requires data on each variable at the beginning and end point of the time period under consideration. A first-difference model with time-varying predictors is structured as follows:

$$(y_{it} - y_{it-1}) = (\mu_t - \mu_{t-1}) + \beta(x_{it} - x_{it-1}) + (\varepsilon_{it} - \varepsilon_{it-1})$$

Subscript *i* represents each unit of analysis (i.e., country), subscript *t* represents the time period, y_{it} is the dependent variable for each country at each time period, μ_t is an intercept that may be different for each time period, and β represents a vector of coefficients. Predictor variables that vary over time are represented by the vector x_{it}, and ε_{it} represents purely random variation at each time point.

We employ difference of logs models in which data for each variable at each time point is logged and then differenced. Each variable, in turn, consists of a relative change score. Difference of logs models effectively estimate the rate of change, expressed as a percent, of the predictor variable on the dependent variable (Firebaugh and Beck 1994; Jackman 1980). In turn, the percentage rate change in the dependent variable is assumed to be a linear function of the percentage rate change in the predictor variable, ceteris paribus.

As opposed to cross-sectional analysis, panel regression is particularly advantageous for evaluating causal propositions as it examines the impact of the independent variables over time, and it is a viable strategy for assessing the effects of structural processes that often take some time to occur (Finkel 1995; Firebaugh and Beck 1994; Liker et al. 1985). First-difference panel analysis, in particular, has the unique advantage of controlling for omitted variable bias in regards to time-invariant (or nearly time-invariant) national characteristics (Allison 2009; Babones 2009; Firebaugh and Beck 1994; Liker et al. 1985). A persistent obstacle in cross-national quantitative research is the frequently unmeasured influence of time-invariant country characteristics given the difficulties in quantifying such disparate considerations (Halaby 2004). Such characteristics can include history, culture, geography, climate, or any other enduring dynamics that may have an effect on the dependent variable and, if unmeasured, can potentially bias the derived regression coefficients.

First-difference panel regression eliminates the impact of time-invariant predictors since their difference scores are, by construction, zero (Allison 2009; Babones 2009; Firebaugh and Beck 1994; Halaby 2004; Kennedy 2008; Liker et al. 1985). In turn, this approach is a viable strategy for dealing with omitted variable bias, even though the time-invariant variables are not actually measured. First-difference models also tend to yield more robust results because potential outliers exert less influence, it avoids out of bounds estimates, and its coefficients have a ready interpretation as the effect of one rate on the other (Firebaugh and Beck 1994). Of note, first-difference models for two time points yield results identical to fixed effects model estimates (Allison 2009).[1]

DEPENDENT VARIABLE

Infant mortality rate (per 1,000 live births) 1990, 2005, 2007 (natural log). Data source: World Bank (2009). This variable measures the probability of a child dying between birth and the age of one, expressed per 1,000 live births.

Main Independent Variable

Urban slum prevalence (% of the total population living in urban slum conditions) 1990, 2005 (natural log). Data source: calculated from data obtained through UN-HABITAT (2008). An urban slum household lacks one or more of the following: access to improved water, access to improved sanitation, sufficient living area, or durability of construction (see Table 1 for more details). As opposed to previous efforts to measure urban slums by examining contiguous settlements exhibiting substandard living conditions, the current methodology focuses on the degree of deprivation relative to the four criteria reiterated above at the household level. This is accomplished through the analysis of an array of household surveys and national census data. See UN-HABITAT (2003a) for more information.

---

[1] Also note there is increasing consensus that a first-difference panel model possesses a number of advantages relative to a lagged dependent variable, or static-score, panel model under most conditions; the latter entails the regression of the dependent variable at a later point in time (t_2) on its value at an earlier point in time (t_1) and on the other independent variables measured at the earlier point in time (t_1). See: Allison (2009), Babones (2009), Firebaugh and Beck (1994), Halaby (2004), Liker et al. (1985).

Additional Independent Variables in the First-Difference Regression Models

Gross domestic product (GDP) per capita (constant 2000 US$) 1990, 2005 (natural log). Data source: World Bank (2009). This variable measures the annual market value of all final goods and services produced domestically relative to the mid-year total population. Economic development as measured by GDP per capita has a strong, direct effect producing lower infant mortality rates (Fay et al. 2005; Filmer and Pritchett 1999; Firebaugh and Beck 1994; Hanmer, Lensink, and White 2003; Lena and London 1993; Moon and Dixon 1985; Moore, Teixeira, and Shiell 2006; Tsai 2006; Wang 2003). Expanding income per capita raises general living standards (Firebaugh and Beck 1994), and it translates into better nutrition, housing, and sanitation, all of which have a beneficial impact on infant mortality rates (Filmer and Pritchett 1999).

Fertility rate, total (births per woman) 1990, 2005 (natural log). Data source: World Bank (2009). This variable is an estimate of the number of children an average women would have if current age-specific fertility rates remained constant during her reproductive years. Fertility rate has been illustrated to have a strong positive effect producing higher infant mortality rates in the developing countries (Wickrama and Lorenz 2002). High fertility levels not only subject women to a greater lifetime risk of maternal mortality but impact the health of infants as the degree of reproductive autonomy women obtain subsequently impacts the control they possess over their own health concerns and that of their children (Wickrama and Lorenz 2002). Such control is rooted in access to various resources and decision-making opportunities (Wickrama and Lorenz 2002). The empowerment of women, in turn, contributes to lower fertility levels even as lower fertility levels reinforce and expand the options women possess in pursuing social well-being concerns, including the health care of infants.

Public health expenditure (% of GDP) 1990, 2005 (natural log). Data source: World Bank (2009). This variable measures governmental investment in healthcare. Many researchers contend infant mortality rates can be reduced through concerted social policy efforts oriented towards the provisioning of key information and health care services broadly throughout society. The efficacy of public health expenditures, however, is a contested issue. Some previous research indeed illustrates public health expenditures are a statistically significant determinant of lower infant mortality rates (Hanmer et al. 2003; Hill and Pebley 1989; Wang 2003). This effect, however, is generally weaker and less robust than level of economic development. Other research fails to find a statistically significant influence of public sector spending on health and infant mortality rates in the developing countries (Filmer and Pritchett 1999; Jorgenson 2004; Jorgenson and Burns 2004; Shandra et al. 2004).

External debt (% of GDP) 1990, 2005 (natural log). Data source: World Bank (2009). This variable includes the sum of short and long-term external debt contracted bilaterally with other states, multilaterally through institutions such as the International Monetary Fund (IMF) and World Bank, and private lending through commercial banks and bank syndicates--expressed as a percent of gross domestic product. Long-term external debt includes: 1) *public* debt guaranteed by the state; 2) *publicly guaranteed* debt in which a private debtor enters into an external (foreign) obligation that is guaranteed by the state; and, 3) *private non-guaranteed* debt in which a private debtor enters into an external obligation that is not guaranteed by the state. In general, the long-term external debt of the developing countries disproportionately consists of public and publicly guaranteed debt entered into by the state or state-owned enterprises.

Many scholars argue the external debt burden impedes the capacity of LDCs to maintain or expand health care delivery to a broad array of the populace as spending on social services becomes increasingly difficult within a context of debt repayment requirements (Bradshaw et al. 1993; Hill and Pebley 1989). Debt service payments are a drain on state income that could alternatively be invested in the upgrading of public services, including housing, and it entrenches export-oriented economic production in order to obtain foreign currency (UN-HABITAT 2003b). Previous research highlights external debt burden exhibits a direct effect shaping higher infant mortality levels in the developing countries (Frey and Field 2000).

Urban population (% of the total population) 1990, 2005 (natural log). Data source: World Bank (2009). We include this variable in the regression analyses in an effort to disentangle the influence of urban slum living conditions from the pace of urbanization, per se, on the dependent variable. It is plausible that rapid urbanization, rather than expansion of urban slums, has a deleterious effect on infant mortality rates in the LDCs.

Overurbanization 1990, 2005 (natural log). Data source: calculated from data obtained through the World Bank (2009). Overurbanization refers to a level of urban social organization deemed excessive relative to concurrent level of economic development, suggesting urban agglomeration without parallel economic development. We adopt the operational definition that is the most frequently employed in the research literature (see: Bradshaw 1985, 1987; Bradshaw and Schafer 2000; Shandra, London, and Williamson 2003; Timberlake and Kentor 1983). This entails the regression of urban population (% of the total population) upon GDP per capita, both measured at the same points in time. The unstandardized residuals or error terms are saved and examined as indicators of relative overurbanization. Low unstandardized residuals signify countries with lower urban social organization than expected given concurrent level of GDP per capita. High residuals indicate countries with higher urbanization than expected given their per capita income level.

Research illustrates overurbanization has a suppressing influence on income per capita within the developing countries (Bradshaw 1985; Bradshaw and Schafer 2000); further, it contributes to expansion of the informal and service sectors of the economy and the production of a surplus urban labor pool that promotes unemployment, underemployment, and low wage levels among unskilled workers (Bradshaw 1985). We include overurbanization in the analyses that follow in an effort to differentiate its potential effect on the dependent variable from that of urban slum prevalence.

Additional Independent Variable Included in the Cross-Sectional Regression Models

Adequate data are unavailable in 1990 for female secondary school enrollment. This precludes the estimation of first-difference models that include this variable. In turn, subsequent to the first-difference model estimates we also report cross-sectional regression models that include urban slum prevalence as the primary predictor of interest, female secondary school enrollment, and each of the control variables outlined above.

Female secondary school gross enrollment ratio (%) 2000-2005. This variable is logged due to evidence of a non-normal distribution. Data source: United Nations Educational, Scientific, and Cultural Organization [UNESCO] (2009). This variable measures the number of females enrolled at the secondary school level expressed as a percent of the total number of females in the relevant age group. Secondary education is generally intended to include the conveyance of basic skills and knowledge and constitutes the end stage of compulsory education. Data refer to any year within this period.

Greater female educational attainment is a strong and robust predictor of lower infant mortality rates (Filmer and Pritchett 1999; Frey and Field 2000; Hanmer et al. 2003; Hobcraft, McDonald, and Rutstein 1984). Caldwell (1990) argues female education enhances not simply access to health services but management and application of the information and services received. He notes educated women tend to engage in greater preventative measures to keep children from becoming sick and more effective and assertive efforts to treat a child after they have fallen ill.

REGRESSION DIAGNOSTICS

We report variance inflation factor (VIF) values in all regression models. There is no well-defined critical VIF value beyond which multicollinearity among predictor variables is a clearly defined problem (Field 1995; Stine 1995). There are, however, symptoms of multicollinearity highlighting potential problems. First, high standard errors are a symptom of multicollinearity and indicate coefficient estimates are imprecise and likely to vary across different samples (Hamilton 1992). Second, a situation wherein the addition or deletion of an independent variable across successive regression models produces substantial changes in the estimated regression coefficients is a common symptom (Hamilton 1992). Third, standardized regression coefficients greater than or less than 1 warn of excessive multicollinearity. None of the regression models in the present study exhibit these classic symptoms.

We utilize Cook's distance and DFBETA values to identify overly influential outlying cases or data points. Any corrections to the dataset due to overly influential outliers are noted in footnotes in the section that follows. Descriptive statistics and bivariate correlations for all variables are included in Tables 2A-5A in the Appendix.

Chapter 5

RESULTS AND DISCUSSION

FIRST-DIFFERENCE PANEL REGRESSION MODELS

The analysis proceeds with the inclusion of urban slum prevalence, the main explanatory variable of interest. We then introduce alternative explanatory measures in a hierarchical manner to evaluate the strength, stability, and statistical significance of urban slum prevalence on infant mortality rates.

Model 1 in Table 2 illustrates urban slum prevalence has a moderately strong, statistically significant effect on infant mortality rates across the 81 developing countries under examination.[1] Approximately 18 percent of the variance in the dependent variable is accounted for by the urban slum prevalence measure. The result highlighted in model 1, moreover, provides empirical evidence that over the period 1990 to 2005 a one percent increase in urban slum prevalence contributes to a .25 percent increase in infant mortality rates, cetiris paribus.

Model 2 in Table 2 highlights economic development as measured by GDP per capita has a moderately strong and statistically significant negative effect on the dependent variable. In turn, a one percent increase in GDP per capita between 1990 and 2005 contributes to a .32 percent decline in infant mortality rates. This is consistent with previous research illustrating per capita income contributes to lower infant mortality rates in the developing

---

[1] F-tests for all regression models are statistically significant at the .001 level and are therefore not reported here.

countries (Fay et al. 2005; Filmer and Pritchett 1999; Firebaugh and Beck 1994; Hanmer et al. 2003; Lena and London 1993; Moon and Dixon 1985; Moore et al. 2006; Tsai 2006; Wang 2003).

Table 2. First-Different Panel Regression: Determinants of Infant Mortality Rate Change, 1990-2005 (ln)

Independent Variables	Model 1	Model 2	Model 3	Model 4	Model 5	Model 6	Model 7
Constant	(.030)	(.035)	(.051)	(.051)	(.050)	(.058)	(.068)
Urban Slum Prevalence Change (% of Total Pop.), 1990-2005 (ln)	.429*** [.251] (.059) *1.000*	.372*** [.217] (.056) *1.026*	.376*** [.220] (.052) *1.026*	.379*** [.221] (.052) *1.027*	.403*** [.236] (.053) *1.060*	.390*** [.228] (.055) *1.133*	.370*** [.216] (.056) *1.199*
GDP Per Capita Change, 1990-2005 (ln)		-.358*** [-.326] (.087) *1.026*	-.242** [-.219] (.088) *1.186*	-.252** [-.229] (.088) *1.194*	-.224* [-.203] (.088) *1.239*	-.231* [-.209] (.090) *1.260*	-.273** [-.248] (.100) *1.555*
Fertility Rate Change, 1990-2005 (ln)			.315*** [.524] (.159) *1.158*	.314*** [.522] (.158) *1.158*	.304*** [.506] (.157) *1.163*	.305*** [.507] (.158) *1.163*	.296*** [.492] (.159) *1.176*
Public Health Expenditure (% of GDP) Change, 1990-2005 (ln)				-.114 [-.095] (.073) *1.009*	-.121 [-.100] (.073) *1.012*	-.127 [-.105] (.074) *1.024*	-.129 [-.106] (.074) *1.025*
External Debt (% of GDP) Change, 1990-2005 (ln)					.140 [.059] (.038) *1.086*	.128 [.053] (.039) *1.150*	.123 [.051] (.039) *1.155*
Urban Population (% of Total Pop.) Change, 1990-2005 (ln)						.052 [.081] (.145) *1.127*	.101 [.158] (.169) *1.517*
Overurbanization Change, 1990-2005 (ln)							-.099 [-.104] (.116) *1.554*
Countries	81	81	81	81	81	81	81
R^2	.184	.309	.395	.408	.426	.428	.435
Adjusted R^2	.174	.292	.371	.377	.388	.382	.380

Note: first number reported is the standardized coefficient, unstandardized coefficients in brackets, standard errors in parentheses, VIFs in italics;

*$p<.05$ **$p<.01$ ***$p<.001$ (two-tailed tests); ln = natural log transformation.

Of particular note, the inclusion of GDP per capita in the regression model tempers but does not substantially reduce the effect of urban slum prevalence on infant mortality rates. The robust influence of the increasing proportion of the total population living in urban slum conditions on growth in infant mortality rates, net the effect of GDP per capita, suggests the influence of the built urban environment is not simply analogous to poverty or lack of economic development; urban slum living conditions illustrate an independent direct effect on infant mortality rates measured at the national level.

Model 3 in Table 2 includes a control for fertility change over the period 1990 to 2005. The results indicate fertility rate has a strong positive effect on infant mortality rates. In turn, the increasing lack of reproductive autonomy produces higher infant mortality rates net the alternative predictors included in model 3. This is consistent with previous research (Wickrama and Lorenz 2002). Also of note, the inclusion of fertility in the regression model tempers the impact of GDP per capita on the dependent variable. This effect, however, remains statistically significant, as does the influence of urban slum prevalence. Overall, the three variables in model 3 account for approximately 39 percent of the variance in the dependent variable.

Model 4 includes consideration of public health expenditures. This measure does not exhibit a statistically significant influence on the dependent variable. This result is at odds with previous research (Hanmer et al. 2003; Hill and Pebley 1989; Wang 2003) but congruent with other research that also fails to find a statistically significant effect on infant mortality rates in the developing countries (Filmer and Pritchett 1999; Jorgenson 2004; Jorgenson and Burns 2004; Shandra et al. 2004).

External debt is included in the regression analysis in model 5, but this measure does not exhibit a statistically significant influence on infant mortality rates net the other explanatory variables included in the model. This is in contrast to previous research illustrating the direct effect of external debt on cross-national infant mortality rates (Frey and Field 2000). It is plausible that the influence of external debt is more appropriately conceptualized as indirect through the promotion of urban slum prevalence. This is an assertion that is untested, but not un-identified (Davis 2006; Rice 2008; Rice and Rice 2009; UN-HABITAT 2003a, 2003b), and may be a valuable focus for future research efforts.

Model 6 in Table 2 includes urban population change. It is plausible that a rapid pace of urbanization rather than urban slum growth per se has a deleterious influence on infant mortality rates. The results presented in model 6, however, do not support this assertion. In turn, urban slum prevalence growth over the period 1990 to 2005 contributes to an increase in infant mortality rates net urbanization.

Model 7 includes a measure of overurbanization. We include this variable to ensure the influence of urban slum prevalence on the dependent variable is not simply a reflection of the impact of overurbanization dynamics, which have been the subject of considerable attention in the research literature. The results highlight urban slum prevalence has an independent direct effect on infant mortality rates net the inclusion of overurbanization, which does not exhibit a statistically significant effect.

Overall the regression models in Table 2 illustrate increasing urban slum prevalence is a significant predictor of increasing infant mortality rates. This positive direct effect, moreover, is robust net the additional statistically significant effects of economic development and fertility rate. The results are suggestive of an urban penalty derived from the inadequate, over-stressed built urban environment. This is consistent with the meta-theoretical assumption derived from social epidemiology asserting the built environment can have physiological consequences and the assertion that health disparities are often rooted in deep-seated, and oppressive, social conditions. Infant mortality is not simply derived from individual-level biological and behavioral risk factors but shaped by the social production of differential exposure to sub-standard urban living conditions as embodied in the formation and expansion of urban slums. It suggests, moreover, that efforts to improve infant morality rates should explicitly confront the urbanization of poverty as embodied in the formation and expansion of urban slum living conditions.

Cross-Sectional Regression Models

Table 3 presents cross-sectional regression models utilizing OLS estimation.[2] The dependent variable is measured in 2007 and all independent variables are measured at an earlier point in time, consistent with the well-

---

[2] Consistent with normative practice in macro-comparative cross-sectional regression analysis, only those variables in Table 3 exhibiting a non-normal distribution are in natural logarithmic form.

known temporal ordering implied in causal analysis. The results reported in Table 3 are intended as a sensitivity check in an effort to further evaluate the impact of urban slum prevalence on infant mortality rates; we include the additional variable measuring female secondary school enrollment which, due to the lack of available data, was absent from the previous panel models.

Model 1 in Table 3 illustrates that urban slum prevalence has a moderately strong and statistically significant effect contributing to higher levels of infant mortality rates among the 81 countries under examination. Approximately 10 percent of the variance in the dependent variable in 2007 is accounted for by this measure.

Model 2 includes GDP per capita in the regression model. The results highlight that economic development has a very strong, statistically significant negative effect on the dependent variable. The influence of urban slum prevalence, moreover, is tempered but remains a moderately strong and statistically significant predictor of higher levels of infant mortality net the inclusion of GDP per capita. Both variables combined account for approximately 75 percent of the variance in the dependent variable.

Model 3 in Table 4 includes consideration of fertility rate. The results highlight that the level of fertility in 2005 has a moderately strong and statistically significant positive effect on the level of infant mortality rates in 2007. Consistent with the panel analysis reported previously, urban slum prevalence, GDP per capita, and fertility all exhibit independent direct effects on infant mortality rates in the developing countries.

Female secondary school enrollment is included in the cross-sectional analysis in models 4-7.[3] The inclusion of female educational enrollment and fertility in the same regression model produces excessive multicollinearity among the explanatory variables, potentially biasing the derived coefficients.[4] In turn, in models 4-7 we exclude fertility rate from the analysis. Of note, previous research suggests fertility may act as a mediating influence whereby female education has an indirect effect on various mortality measures, including infant mortality (Wickrama and Lorenz 2002). That is, expanding female educational achievement has a strong negative effect on the prevailing fertility rate (Gallagher, Stokes, and Anderson 1996)

---

[3] Tanzania was excluded from models 4-7 in Table 3 due to its excessively high Cook's D value.

[4] The Pearson bivariate correlation coefficient between female secondary school enrollment and fertility rate is -.877 and is statistically significant at the .001 level.

which then has a strong negative effect on infant mortality (Wickrama and Lorenz 2002).

Table 3. Cross-Sectional Regression: Determinants of Infant Mortality Rate 2007 (ln)

Independent Variables	Model 1	Model 2	Model 3	Model 4	Model 5	Model 6	Model 7
Constant	(.160)	(.273)	(.503)	(.254)	(.442)	(.560)	(.465)
Urban Slum Prevalence (% of Total Population) 2005	.320** [.018] (.006) *1.000*	.260*** [.014] (.003) *1.005*	.174*** [.010] (.003) *1.150*	.207*** [.012] (.003) *1.064*	.208*** [.012] (.003) *1.083*	.209*** [.012] (.003) *1.316*	.209*** [.012] (.003) *1.316*
GDP Per Capita 2005 (ln)		- .812*** [-.547] (.038) *1.005*	- .514*** [-.346] (.055) *2.728*	- .471*** [-.317] (.062) *3.244*	- .458*** [-.309] (.066) *3.616*	- .454*** [-.306] (.088) *6.258*	- .458*** [-.309] (.067) *3.618*
Fertility Rate 2005			.390*** [.197] (.043) *2.941*				
Female Secondary School Enrollment (%) 2000-2005 (ln)				- .421*** [-.464] (.103) *3.333*	- .430*** [-.474] (.105) *3.382*	- .430*** [-.473] (.105) *3.391*	- .430*** [-.473] (.105) *3.391*
Public Health Expenditures (% of GDP) 2005 (ln)					.030 [.040] (.075) *1.155*	.030 [.040] (.076) *1.162*	.030 [.040] (.076) *1.162*

Independent Variables	Model 1	Model 2	Model 3	Model 4	Model 5	Model 6	Model 7
Constant	(.160)	(.273)	(.503)	(.254)	(.442)	(.560)	(.465)
External Debt (% of GNP) 2005 (ln)					.033 [.037] (.065) *1.243*	.034 [.038] (.067) *1.325*	.034 [.038] (.067) *1.325*
Urban Population (% of Total Population) 2005						-.005 [.000] (.004) *3.832*	
Overurbanization 2005							-.003 [.000] (.004) *1.307*
Countries	81	81	81	78	78	78	78
R^2	.102	.758	.810	.806	.808	.808	.808
Adjusted R^2	.091	.752	.802	.798	.794	.791	.791

Note: first number reported is the standardized coefficient, unstandardized coefficients in brackets, standard errors in parentheses, VIFs in italics; *p<.05 **p<.01 ***p<.001 (two-tailed tests); ln = natural log transformation.

The results presented in model 4 illustrate female secondary school enrollment has a strong and statistically significant negative effect on infant mortality rates. In turn, as the level of female secondary educational enrollment increases infant mortality rates decrease. This is consistent with previous research (Filmer and Pritchett 1999; Frey and Field 2000; Hanmer et al. 2003; Hobcraft et al.1984) and supports the assertion that the educational empowerment of women has a direct influence on infant mortality rates net level of economic development. Also of note, urban slum prevalence remains a statistically significant predictor of infant mortality rates in model 4 net the inclusion and strong influence of female secondary school enrollment as well as the robust negative effect of GDP per capita. These three variables account for approximately 80 percent of the variance in the dependent variable in model 4.

Models 5-7 in Table 3 include additional control variables presented in order to further assess the strength and stability of urban slum prevalence on the dependent variable. Consistent with the results presented previously in the panel regression models, none of the variables introduced in models 5-7 have a statistically significant effect on infant mortality rates; further, their inclusion in the analysis does not substantively alter the influence of urban slum prevalence on the dependent variable.[1]

---

[1] We incorporated into the cross-sectional regression analysis additional explanatory variables not reported here. None were statistically significant predictors of infant mortality nor did their inclusion substantively alter the results reported in Table 3. First, we included skilled attendants at delivery (% of births) as an indicator of health services. Second, we included contraceptive prevalence (%) among married women ages 15-49.

Chapter 6

CONCLUSION

The growth of urban slums in the LDCs is a structural trend producing concentrated disadvantage (Vlahov et al. 2007) recognizable in the overcrowding and substandard living conditions enveloping nearly one billion people worldwide. Further, their historically unprecedented rise threatens to undercut the presumed public health advantages of urban life in ways many researchers have yet to fully consider.

The intent of the present study is to empirically examine the potential social production of infant mortality by focusing on the direct influence of urban slum prevalence or proportion of the total population living in urban slum conditions among the 81 developing countries with available data. This analytical focus is grounded in the meta-theoretical assumption derived from social epidemiology suggesting the built environment is not simply a container for social-organizational dynamics but has independent effects on physiological processes and is thus central to prevailing patterns of health and illness. Disparities in health and illness often follow from contextual social determinants shaping variance in risk encountered by differing segments of a population. Such patterns, in turn, constitute "biological reflections of social fault lines" whereby disease distribution is forged through relative power, privilege, and inequality (Farmer 1999: 5; Krieger 2001a; Krieger and Zierler 1996).

Empirical results derived from first-difference panel regression illustrates increasing urban slum prevalence between 1990 and 2005 has a robust effect producing higher levels of infant mortality over the period among the 81 developing countries under examination. This result obtains net the statistically significant beneficial effects of economic development as measured by GDP per capita and the robust deleterious impact of fertility rate. The results provide empirical evidence the built urban environment has a direct effect on infant mortality rates measured at the national level. It lends support to the assertion that there is an observable urban penalty in terms of infant mortality rates derived from the general social and economic exclusion and substandard living conditions characteristic of urban slums in the developing countries. Cross-sectional regression results, in addition, also illustrate urban slum prevalence has a statistically significant influence producing higher levels of infant mortality rates. Of note, this result is robust net the strong, statistically significant effect of female secondary school enrollment, which contributes to lower levels of infant mortality rates.

Consistent with the identification of key social determinants of health, the results demonstrate infant mortality rates in the developing countries are, in part, socially produced through the growth of urban slum living conditions. This lends credence to Krieger's (2001b: 899) assertion: "Context and level matter: poor people living in poor neighborhoods are likely to have poorer health than equally poor people living in more affluent neighborhoods." This is an assertion Engels (1968 [1845]) proffered more than 150 years ago in his examination of the living conditions of the English working class but bears repeating in relation to the burgeoning urban slums of the developing countries. Context matters--particularly for marginalized and vulnerable segments of a population.

Epidemiological studies have greatly contributed to the identification of the individual-level risk factors shaping the incidence of morbidity and mortality, but a renewed emphasis on the identification of "basic social conditions" is crucial to delineating the contextual determinants that further constitute fundamental causes of health or illness (Link and Phelan 1995: 80, 1996). As Gieryn (2000) notes, the physicality of "place" has a tendency to *emplace* or give form to difference, inequality, and marginalization within society. Buildings both stabilize social life (Gieryn 2002) and as cultural artifacts are a reflection of social and economic priorities and prevailing power structures (Baldry 1999).

Evidence that urban slum prevalence has an impact on population-level measures of infant mortality forces consideration of the need for *preventative* in addition to simply *curative* health care efforts in the developing countries. A preventative focus entails the evaluation of the underlying social, built, and biophysical environmental factors shaping morbidity and mortality whereas a curative approach emphasizes specific medical interventions employed to combat morbidity as it arises (Ehiri and Prowse 1999; Hill and Pebley 1989). A long-standing debate concerns the appropriate policies to pursue within the developing countries given the scarce resources available at any given point in time. As Ehiri and Prowse (1999) note, the curative approach has been successful in improving public health in the developing countries, but insufficient consideration of broader contextual dynamics makes it is difficult to sustain progress over the long term.

Few studies from a macro-comparative perspective explicitly focus on the factors promoting and constraining urban slum prevalence growth in the developing countries. In turn, future research efforts that examine in more detail such concerns would constitute an important contribution to existing knowledge regarding the factors that indirectly shape the social production of infant mortality rates. Moreover, an exclusively individual-level, "desocialized" approach, as is common within the biomedical model, impedes conceptualization of the influence of the built urban environment on infant mortality rates and, potentially, increasing challenges to human health more broadly as a consequence of the increasing formation and expansion of urban slums in the developing countries.

REFERENCES

Agarwal, Siddharth & Taneja, Shivani (2005). "All Slums are Not Equal: Child Health Conditions among the Urban Poor." *Indian Pediatrics*, *42*, 233-244.

Allison, Paul, D. (2009). *Fixed Effects Regression Models*. Los Angeles: Sage Publications.

Awasthi, Shally & Agarwal, Siddharth (2003). "Determinants of Childhood Mortality and Morbidity in Urban Slums in India." *Indian Pediatrics*, *40*, 1145-1161.

Babones, Salvatore J. (2009). "Modeling Error in Quantitative Macro-Comparative Research." *Journal of World-Systems Research, 15(1)*, 86-114.

Baldry, Chris. (1999). "'Space—The Final Frontier.'" *Sociology*, *33(3)*, 535-553.

Bartlett, Sheridan. (2003). "Water, Sanitation, and Urban Children: The Need to Go Beyond 'Improved' Provision." *Environment and Urbanization*, *15(2)*, 57-70.

Berkman, Lisa, F. & Kawachi, Ichiro (2000). "A Historical Framework for Social Epidemiology." Pp. 3-12 in *Social Epidemiology*, edited by Lisa F. Berkman and Ichiro Kawachi. NY: Oxford University Press.

Bolay, Jean-Claude. (2006). "Slums and Urban Development: Questions on Society and Globalization." *The European Journal of Development Research*, *18(2)*, 284-298.

Bradshaw, York, W. (1985). "Overurbanization and Underdevelopment in Sub-Saharan Africa: A Cross-National Study." *Studies in Comparative International Development*, *20(3)*, 74-101.

Bradshaw, York, W. (1987). "Urbanization and Underdevelopment: A Global Study of Modernization, Urban Bias, and Economic Dependency." *American Sociological Review, 52*, 224-239.

Bradshaw, York, W. (1993). Rita Noonan, Laura Gash, and Claudia Buchmann Sershen. "Borrowing Against the Future: Children and Third World Indebtedness." *Social Forces,, 71(3)*, 629-656.

Bradshaw, York, W. & Schafer Mark, J. (2000). "Urbanization and Development: The Emergence of International Nongovernmental Organizations amid Declining States." *Sociological Perspectives, 43(1)*, 97-116.

Brown, Valerie, J. (2003). "Give Me Shelter: The Global Housing Crisis." *Environmental Health Perspectives, 111(2)*, A92-A99.

Caldwell, John, C. (1990). "Cultural and Social Factors Influencing Mortality Levels in Developing Countries." *The ANNALS of the American Academy of Political and Social Science, 510(1)*, 44-59.

Cassel, John. (1964). "Social Science Theory as a Source of Hypotheses in Epidemiological Research." *American Journal of Public Health, 54(9)*, 1482-1488.

Cohen, Barney. (2006). "Urbanization in Developing Countries: Current Trends, Future Projections, and Key Challenges for Sustainability." *Technology in Society*, 28: 63-80.

Cwikel, Julie. *Social Epidemiology: Strategies for Public Health Activism.* NY: Columbia University Press.

Davis, Mike. (2006). *Planet of Slums*. New York: Verso.

Dunlap, Riley E. & Catton William, R. Jr. (1979). "Environmental Sociology." *Annual Review of Sociology, 5*, 243-273.

Dunlap, Riley, E., Michelson, William & Stalker, Glenn (2001). "Environmental Sociology: An Introduction" 1-32 in *Handbook of Environmental Sociology*, edited by Riley E. Dunlap and William Michelson. Westport, CT: Greenwood Press.

Ehiri, John, E. & Prowse Julie, M. (1999). "Child Health Promotion in Developing Countries: The Case for Integration of Environmental and Social Interventions?" *Health Policy and Planning, 14(1)*, 1-10.

Engels, Friedrich. (1968). [1845]. *The Condition of the Working Class in England.* Translated and Edited by W.O. Henderson and W.H. Chaloner. Stanford, CA: Stanford University Press.

Fay, Marianne, Danny Leipziger, Quentin Wodon & Tito Yepes. (2005). "Achieving Child-Health-Related Millennium Development Goals: The Role of Infrastructure." *World Development, 33(8)*, 1267-1284.

Farmer, Paul. (1999). *Infections and Inequalities: The Modern Plagues*. Berkeley, CA: The University of California Press.

Farmer, Paul. (2004). "An Anthropology of Structural Violence." *Current Anthropology*, *45(3)*, 305-325.

Farmer, Paul, Bruce Nizeye, Stulac, Sara & Keshavjee, Salmaan (2006). "Structural Violence and Clinical Medicine." *PLoS Medicine*, *3(10)*, 1686-1691.

Fernandez, Armida, Mondkar, Jayshree & Mathai, Sheila (2003). "Urban Slum-Specific Issues in Neonatal Survival." *Indian Pediatrics*, *40*, 1161-1166.

Field, Andy. (2005). *Discovering Statistics Using SPSS*. 2nd Edition. *Thousand Oaks*, CA: Sage Publications.

Filmer, Deon & Pritchett, Lant (1999). "The Impact of Public Spending on Health: Does Money Matter?" *Social Science & Medicine*, *49*, 1309-1323.

Finkel, Steven E. (1995). Causal Analysis with Panel Data. *Thousand Oaks,* CA: Sage.

Firebaugh, Glenn & Beck, Frank D. (1994). "Does Economic Growth Benefit the Masses? Growth, Dependence, and Welfare in the Third World." *American Sociological Review*, *59*, 631-653.

Fitzpatrick, Kevin & LaGory, Mark (2000). *Unhealthy Places: The Ecology of Risk in the Urban Landscape*. NY: Routledge.

Fotso, Jean-Christophe, Ezeh Alex Chika, Madise Nyovani Janet & Ciera, James (2007). "Progress Towards the Child Mortality Millennium Development Goal in Urban Sub-Saharan Africa: The Dynamics of Population Growth, Immunization, and Access to Clean Water." *BMC Public Health*, *7*, 218.

Frey, R. Scott & Carolyn Field. (2000). "The Determinants of Infant Mortality in the Less Developed Countries: A Cross-National Test of Five Theories." *Social Indicators Research*, *52*, 215-234.

Gallagher, Sally, K., Stokes, Randall, G. & Anderson, Andy, B. (1996). "Economic Disarticulation and Fertility in Less Developed Nations." *The Sociological Quarterly*, *37(2)*, 227-244.

Galtung, Johan. (1969). "Violence, Peace, and Peace Research." *Journal of Peace Research*, *6(3)*, 167-191.

Galtung, Johan. (1990). "Cultural Violence." *Journal of Peace Research*, *27(3)*, 291-305.

Ghosh, Shanti & Shah, Dheeraj (2004). "Nutritional Problems in Urban Slum Children." *Indian Pediatrics*, *41*, 682-696.

Gieryn, Thomas F. (2000). "A Space for Place in Sociology." *Annual Review of Sociology, 26*, 463-496.

Gieryn, Thomas F. (2002). "What Buildings Do." *Theory and Society, 31*, 35-74.

Gulati, J. K. & Jaswal, S. (1998). "Maternal and Child Health Care in Slums of Ludhiana City." *Indian Journal of Maternal and Child Health, 9(1)*, 48-51.

Halaby, Charles, N. (2004). "Panel Models in Sociological Research: Theory into Practice." *Annual Review of Sociology, 30*, 507-544.

Hamilton, Lawrence C. (1992). *Regression with Graphics: A Second Course in Applied Statistics*. Belmont, CA: Wadsworth, Inc.

Hanmer Lucia, Lensink Robert & White, Howard (2003). "Infant and Child Mortality in Developing Countries: Analysing the Data for Robust Determinants." *The Journal of Development Studies, 40(1)*, 101-118.

Hill, Kenneth & Anne R. Pebley. (1989). "Child Mortality in the Developing World." *Population and Development Review, 15(4)*, 657-687.

Hobcraft, J. N., McDonald, J. W. & Rutstein, S. O. (1984). "Socio-Economic Factors in Infant and Child Mortality: A Cross-National Comparison." *Population Studies, 38*, 193-223.

Hoque, Ashraful & Selwyn Beatrice, J. (1996). "Birth Practice Patterns in Urban Slums of Dhaka, Bangladesh." *Women & Health, 24(1)*, 41-58.

Jackman, Robert, W. (1980). "A Note on the Measurement of Growth Rates in Cross-National Research." *American Journal of Sociology, 86(3)*, 604-617.

Jorgenson, Andrew K. (2004). Global Inequality, Water Pollution, and Infant Mortality. *The Social Science Journal, 41*, 279-288.

Jorgenson, Andrew K. & Burns, Thomas J. (2004). "Globalization, the Environment, and Infant Mortality: A Cross-National Study." *Humboldt Journal of Social Relations, 28(1)*, 7-52.

Kennedy, Peter. (2008). *A Guide to Econometrics* (6th edition). Malden: Blackwell Publishing.

Kilmartin, Leslie. (2001). "Designing the Built Environment." Pp. 167-191 in *Handbook of Environmental Sociology*, edited by Riley E. Dunlap and William Michelson. Westport, CT: Greenwood Press.

Krieger, Nancy. (1999). "Embodying Inequality: A Review of Concepts, Measures, and Methods for Studying Health Consequences of Discrimination." *International Journal of Health Services, 29(2)*, 295-352.

Krieger, Nancy. (2000). "Epidemiology and Social Sciences: Towards a Critical Reengagement in the 21st Century." *Epidemiologic Reviews, 22(1)*, 155-163.

Krieger, Nancy. (2001a). "Theories for Social Epidemiology in the 21st Century: An Ecosocial Perspective." *International Journal of Epidemiology, 30(4)*, 668-677.

Krieger, Nancy. (2001b). "Historical Roots of Social Epidemiology: Socioeconomic Gradients in Health and Contextual Analysis." *International Journal of Epidemiology*, 30: 899-900.

Krieger, Nancy & Sally Zierler. (1996). "What Explains the Public's Health—A Call for Epidemiologic Theory." *Epidemiology, 7(1)*, 107-109.

Lena, Hugh, F. & Bruce London. (1993). "The Political and Economic Determinants of Health Outcomes: A Cross-National Analysis." *International Journal of Health Services*, 23(3): 585-602.

Liker, Jeffrey, K., Augustyniak, Sue & Duncan Greg, J. (1985). "Panel Data and Models of Change: A Comparison of First Difference and Conventional Two-Wave Models." *Social Science Research, 14*, 80-101.

Link, Bruce G. & Phelan Jo, C. (1995). "Social Conditions as Fundamental Causes of Disease." *Journal of Health and Social Behavior*, Extra Issue: 80-94.

Link, Bruce, G. & Phelan, Jo, C. (1996). "Understanding Sociodemographic Differences in Health—The Role of Fundamental Social Causes." *American Journal of Public Health*, 86(4): 471-473.

Macintyre, Sally & Ellaway, Anne (2000). "Ecological Approaches: Rediscovering the Role of the Physical and Social Environment." 332-348 in *Social Epidemiology*, edited by Lisa F. Berkman and Ichiro Kawachi. NY: Oxford University Press.

McKinlay, John, B. (1981). "A Case for Refocusing Upstream: The Political Economy of Illness." Pp. 613-633 in *The Sociology of Health and Illness: Critical Perspectives*, edited by Peter Conrad and Rochelle Kern. NY: St. Martin's Press.

Moon, Bruce, E. & Dixon, William, J. (1985). "Politics, the State, and Basic Human Needs: A Cross-National Study." *American Journal of Political Science, 29(4)*, 661-694.

Moore, Spencer, Teixeira, Ana C. & Shiell, Alan (2006). "The Health of Nations in a Global Context: Trade, Global Stratification, and Infant Mortality Rates." *Social Science & Medicine*, 63: 165-178.

Oakes, J. Michael & Kaufman, Jay S. (2006). "Introduction: Advancing Methods in Social Epidemiology." Pp. 3-20 in *Methods in Social Epidemiology: Research Design and Methods*, edited by J. Michael Oakes and Jay S. Kaufman. San Francisco, CA: Jossey-Bass.

Rahi Manju, Taneja, D. K. Misra Amrita, Mathur, N. B. & Badhan, Suresh (2006). "Newborn Care Practices in an Urban Slum of Delhi." *Indian Journal of Medical Sciences*, 60(12): 506-513.

Rice, James. (2008). "The Urbanization of Poverty and Urban Slum Prevalence: The Impact of the Built Environment on Population-Level Patterns of Social Well-Being in the Less Developed Countries." 205-234 in *Research in the Sociology of Health Care*. Volume 26, *Care for Major Health Problems and Population Health Concerns: Impacts on Patients, Providers, and Policy*, edited by Jennie Jacobs Kronenfeld. Amsterdam, The Netherlands: Elsevier.

Rice, James & Rice, Julie Steinkopf (2009). "The Concentration of Disadvantage and the Rise of an Urban Penalty: Urban Slum Prevalence and the Social Production of Health Inequalities in the Developing Countries." *International Journal of Health Services*, *39(4)*, 749-770.

Satterthwaite, David. (1993). "The Impact on Health of Urban Environments." *Environment and Urbanization*, *5(2)*, 87-111.

Sclar Elliott, Garau, Pietro & Carolini, Gabriella (2005). "The 21st Century Health Challenge of Slums and Cities." *The Lancet*, March 5, *365*, 901-903.

Shandra, John M., Bruce London & Williamson, John B. (2003). "Environmental Degradation, Environmental Sustainability, and Overurbanization in the Developing World: A Quantitative, Cross-National Analysis." *Sociological Perspectives*, *46(3)*, 309-329.

Shandra, J., Nobles, J., London, B. & Williamson, J. (2004). "Dependency, Democracy, and Infant Mortality: A Quantitative, Cross-National Analysis of Less Developed Countries." *Social Science & Medicine* 59:321-333.

Stine, Robert A. (1995). Graphical Interpretation of Variance Inflation Factors. *The American Statistician*, *49(1)*, 53-56.

Timberlake, Michael & Jeffrey Kentor. (1983). "Economic Dependence, Overurbanization, and Economic Growth: A Study of Less Developed Countries." *The Sociological Quarterly*, *24*, 489-507.

Tsai, Ming-Chang. (2006). "Does Political Democracy Enhance Human Development in Developing Countries? A Cross-National Analysis." *American Journal of Economics and Sociology*, *65(2)*, 233-268.

Turshen, Meredeth. (1977). "The Political Ecology of Disease." *Review of Radical Political Economics, 9(1)*, 45-60.

United Nations Development Programme [UNDP]. (2006). *Human Development Report.* United Nations Development Programme. NY: Oxford University Press.

United Nations Educational, Scientific, and Cultural Organization Institute for Statistics [UNESCO]. 2009. *World Education Indicators.* Paris: UNESCO. Available on-line at: http://www.uis.unesco.org.

United Nations Human Settlements Programme [UN-HABITAT]. (2003a). *Slums of the World: The Face of Urban Poverty in the New Millennium?* London: Earthscan. Available: www.unhabitat.org.

United Nations Human Settlements Programme [UN-HABITAT]. (2003b). *The Challenge of Slums: Global Report on Human Settlements 2003.* London: Earthscan. Available: www.unhabitat.org.

United Nations Human Settlements Programme [UN-HABITAT]. (2006). *State of the World's Cities Report 2006/7.* London: Earthscan. Available: www.unhabitat.org.

United Nations Human Settlements Programme [UN-HABITAT]. (2007a). *Slums: Some Definitions.* Available: www.unhabitat.org. Accessed May.

United Nations Human Settlements Programme [UN-HABITAT]. (2007b). *The Urban Penalty: The Poor Die Young.* Available: www.unhabitat.org. Accessed May.

United Nations Human Settlements Programme [UN-HABITAT]. (2008). UrbanInfo Database. Accessed July, 2009. Available: http://www.devinfo.info/urbaninfo/.

United Nations Population Fund [UNFPA]. (2007). *State of World Population.* Available on-line at: www.unfpa.org.

Vaid, A., Mammen, A., Primrose, B. & Kang, G. (2007). "Infant Mortality in an Urban Slum." *Indian Journal of Pediatrics, 74*, 449-453.

Vlahov, David, Nicholas Freudenberg, Fernando Proietti, Danielle Ompad, Andrew Quinn, Vijay Nandi, and Sandro Galea. 2007. "Urban as a Determinant of Health." *Journal of Urban Health: Bulletin of the New York Academy of Medicine, 84(1)*, i16-i26.

Wagstaff, Adam, Bustreo, Flavia, Bryce, Jennifer & Claeson, Mariam (2004). "Child Health: Reaching the Poor." *American Journal of Public Health, 94(5)*, 726-736.

Waitzkin, Howard. (1981). "The Social Origins of Illness: A Neglected History." *International Journal of Health Services, 11(1)*, 77-103.

Wang, Limin. (2003). "Determinants of Child Mortality in LDCs: Empirical Findings from Demographic and Health Surveys." *Health Policy, 65*, 277-299.

Wickrama, K. A. S. & Lorenz Frederick, O. (2002). "Women's Status, Fertility Decline, and Women's Health in Developing Countries: Direct and Indirect Influences of Social Status on Health." *Rural Sociology, 67(2)*, 255-277.

World Bank. (2006). *Historical Income Classifications*. Retrieved October, 2006 (http://www.worldbank.org). Washington, DC: World Bank.

World Bank. (2009). *World Development Indicators Online*. Washington, DC: The World Bank. Available on-line at: http://www.worldbank.org.

Yankauer, Alfred, Jr. (1950). "The Relationship of Fetal and Infant Mortality to Residential Segregation: An Inquiry into Social Epidemiology." *American Sociological Review, 15*, 644-648.

APPENDIX

Table 1A. Countries included in the regression analyses (N = 81)

Algeria	Ethiopia	Nicaragua
Angola	Gambia	Niger
Argentina	Ghana	Nigeria
Bangladesh	Guatemala	Oman
Belize	Guinea	Pakistan
Benin	Guinea-Bissau	Panama
Bhutan	Guyana	Paraguay
Bolivia	Haiti	Peru
Botswana	Honduras	Philippines
Brazil	India	Rwanda
Burkina Faso	Indonesia	Senegal
Burundi	Iran	Sierra Leone
Cambodia	Jamaica	Sri Lanka
Cameroon	Jordan	Sudan
Central African Republic	Kenya	Syria
Chad	Laos	Tanzania
Chile	Lebanon	Thailand
China	Lesotho	Togo
Colombia	Madagascar	Tunisia
Congo	Malawi	Turkey
Congo, Democratic Rep. of	Malaysia	Uganda
Costa Rica	Mali	Uruguay
Cote d'Ivoire	Mauritania	Venezuela
Dominican Republic	Mexico	Viet Nam
Ecuador	Morocco	Yemen
Egypt	Mozambique	Zambia
El Salvador	Nepal	Zimbabwe

Table 2A. Descriptive summary of the variables included in the first-difference regression analysis

Variable	N	Min	Max	Mean	Std. Dev.	Skew
Infant Mortality Rate Change, 1990-2005	81	-1.18	.21	-.38	.29	-.344
Urban Slum Prevalence Change, 1990-2005	81	-2.92	1.12	.11	.49	-3.53
GDP Per Capita Change, 1990-2005	81	-.82	1.31	.24	.32	-.192
Fertility Rate Change, 1990-2005	81	-.85	.00	-.29	.17	-.966
Public Health Expenditure Change, 1990-2005	81	-1.29	.78	-.04	.35	-.581
External Debt Change, 1990-2005	81	-2.34	1.24	-.39	.69	-.189
Urban Population Change, 1990-2005	81	-.13	1.27	.19	.19	2.59
Overurbanization Change, 1990-2005	81	-.36	1.20	.39	.27	.580

Note: all variables have been logged and differenced.

Table 3A. Correlation matrix of the variables included in the first-difference regression analysis

		1.	2.	3.	4.	5.	6.	7.
Infant Mortality Rate Change, 1990-2005	1.	---						
Urban Slum Prevalence Change, 1990-2005	2.	.429***	---					
GDP Per Capita Change, 1990-2005	3.	-.418***	-.160	---				
Fertility Rate Change, 1990-2005	4.	.421***	.046	-.369***	---			
Public Health Expenditure Change, 1990-2005	5.	-.068	.039	-.093	.027	---		
External Debt Change, 1990-2005	6.	.165	-.137	-.206	.138	.064	---	
Urban Population Change, 1990-2005	7.	.127	.204	.039	-.012	.116	.182	---
Overurbanization Change, 1990-2005	8.	.049	-.031	-.338**	.049	.065	.142	.431***

Note: all variables have been logged and differenced; *$p<.05$ **$p<.01$ ***$p<.001$ (two-tailed tests).

Table 4A. Descriptive summary of the variables included in the cross-sectional regression analysis

Variable	N	Min	Max	Mean	Std. Dev.	Skew
Infant Mortality Rate, 2007 (ln)	81	1.79	5.04	3.72	.79	-.346
Urban Slum Prevalence, 2005	81	.20	62.4	23	14.2	.482
GDP Per Capita, 2005 (ln)	81	4.49	9.20	6.75	1.17	-.194
Fertility Rate, 2005	81	1.81	7.08	3.87	1.56	.497
Female Secondary Education, 2000-2005 (ln)	78	1.61	4.71	3.73	.75	-7.07
Public Health Expenditure, 2005 (ln)	81	-.92	2.16	.82	.58	-.238
External Debt, 2005 (ln)	81	1.59	5.48	3.92	.69	-.441
Urban Population, 2005	81	10	93.4	45.9	21.8	.323
Overurbanization, 2005	81	-37.5	23.2	.000	12.8	-.514

ln = natural log transformation.

Table 5A. Correlation matrix of variables contained in the descriptive and regression analyses

		1.	2.	3.	4.	5.	6.	7.	8.
Infant Mortality Rate, 2007 (ln)	**1.**	---							
Urban Slum Prevalence, 2005	**2.**	.320**	---						
GDP Per Capita, 2005 (ln)	**3.**	-.831***	-.074	---					
Fertility Rate, 2005	**4.**	.840***	.278**	-.782***	---				
Female Secondary Education, 2000-2005 (ln)	**5.**	-.824***	-.194	.810***	-.877***	---			
Public Health Expenditure, 2005 (ln)	**6.**	-.280**	-.139	.300**	-.221*	.293**	---		
External Debt, 2005 (ln)	**7.**	.373***	.060	-.413***	.371***	-.315**	-.037	---	
Urban Population, 2005	**8.**	-.615***	.181	.811***	-.546***	.656***	.266**	-.203	---
Overurbanization, 2005	**9.**	.120	.412***	.000	.151	.011	.039	.226*	.585***

Note: *p<.05 **p<.01 ***p<.001 (two-tailed tests); ln = natural log transformation

INDEX

A

B

C

D

E

F

G

H

I

V

W

Y

Z